The

Sirtfood Diet

The Ultimate Guide to Lose Weight, Burn Fat, Get Lean and Feel Good!

Table of Contents

Introduction

The Sirtfood Diet, also called the skinny gene-diet, is the result of the studies of the two nutritionists Aidan Goggings and Glenn Matten. Their food program, published in a volume that explains its principles and functioning, has attracted the attention of VIPs and sportsmen. Its effectiveness is based on the consumption of foods that stimulate sirtuins. As the creators of the diet of the moment explain, it is a family of genes present in each of us. They affect the ability to burn fat in addition to mood and the mechanisms that regulate longevity. It is no coincidence that they are also called "super metabolic regulators." Recent studies have shown that there are a number of foods that can stimulate sirtuins. Their consumption would, therefore, allow them to activate the metabolism and lose weight without having to undergo extreme diets.

What makes the Sirtfood Diet different from the others is its "inclusion" philosophy. In fact, it is not based on the total or partial exclusion of some foods from your diet. Rather, it suggests which foods should be added to lose weight more easily. In this way, you will no longer have to undergo excessive deprivation or exhausting willpower. And you won't have to resort to expensive supplements or products with mysterious components. By eating a balanced diet and supporting it, if desired, with proper physical activity, according to the two nutritionists, you can lose about 3.5 kilos in a week.

After the discovery in 2003, the enthusiasm for the benefits of Sort's food skyrocketed. Studies revealed that these foods don't just mimic the effects of calorie restriction. They also act as super regulators of the entire metabolism: they burn fat, increase muscle mass, and improve the health of our cells. The world of medical research was close to the most important nutritional discovery of the century. Unfortunately, a mistake was made: the pharmaceutical industry invested hundreds of millions of pounds in an attempt to turn Sirt foods into a sort of miracle pill, and the diet took a back seat. The Sirtfood Diet, however, does not share this pharmaceutical approach, which seeks to concentrate the benefits of these complex nutrients of plant origin into a single drug. Instead of waiting for the pharmaceutical industry to transform the nutrients of the foods we eat into a miraculous product which may not work anyway, the Sirtfood Diet consists of eating these substances in their natural form that of food, to take full advantage of them. This is the basis of the pilot experiment of the Sirtfood Diet, with which the creators intended to create a diet containing the richest sources of Sirt foods and observe their effects.

During their studies, Glen Matten and Aidan Goggins discovered that the best Sirt foods are consumed regularly by populations who boast the lowest incidence of diseases and obesity in the world.

The Kuna Indians, in the American continent, seem immune from hypertension and with very low levels of obesity, diabetes, cancer, and early death thanks to the intake of cocoa, excellent Sirt food. In Okinawa, Japan, Sirt food, dry physique, and longevity go hand in hand. In India, the passion for spicy foods, especially turmeric, gives good results in the fight against cancer. And in the traditional Mediterranean diet, which the rest of the western world envies, obesity is contained, and chronic diseases are the exception, not the norm. Extra virgin olive oil, wild green leafy vegetables, dried fruit, berries, red wine, dates, and aromatic herbs are all effective Sirt foods, and they are all present in the Mediterranean diet. The scientific world has had to surrender to the evidence: it seems that the Mediterranean diet is more effective than reducing calories to lose weight and more effective than drugs to eliminate diseases.

The good news is that you don't have to be a top athlete, and not even sporty, to enjoy the same benefits. We took advantage of everything we learned about Sirt foods thanks to the pilot study by KX and the work done with sportsmen, and we adapted it to create a diet suitable for anyone who wants to lose weight while improving health.

It is not necessary to practice unsustainable fasting or to undergo endless sessions in the gym although, of course, practicing a little physical activity would be good for you. It is not an

expensive diet nor will it waste your time, and all the foods recommended in the diet are readily available. The only accessory
you will need is an extractor or centrifuge. Unlike other diets,
which tell you what to eliminate, this diet tells you what to eat.

Chapter 1 - Which Are the Sirtfoods

The basis of the sirtuin diet can be explained in simple terms or in complex ways. It is important to also know why these sirtuin rich foods help to help you maintain fidelity to your diet plan. Otherwise, you may throw something in your meal with less nutrition that would defeat the purpose of planning for one rich in sirtuins. Most importantly, this is not a dietary fad, and as you will see, there is much wisdom contained in how humans have used natural foods even for medicinal purposes, over thousands of years.

To understand how the Sirtfood diet works, and why these particular foods are necessary, we will look at the role they play in the human body.

Sirtuin activity was first researched in yeast, where a mutation caused an extension in the yeast's lifespan. Sirtuins were also shown to slow aging in laboratory mice, fruit flies, and nematodes. As research on Sirtuins proved to transfer to mammals, they were examined for their use in diet and slowing the aging process. The sirtuins in humans are different in the typing but they essentially work in the same ways and reasons.

There are seven "members" that make up the sirtuin family. It is believed that sirtuins play a big role in regulating certain functions of cells including proliferation reproduction and growth of cells, apoptosis death of cells. They promote survival and resist stress to increase longevity.

They are also seen to block neurodegeneration. They conduct their housekeeping functions by cleaning out toxic proteins and supporting the brain's ability to change and adapt to different conditions, or to recuperate. As part of this they also help reduce chronic inflammation, and reduce something called oxidative stress. Oxidative stress is when there are too many cell-damaging free radicals circulating in the body, and the body cannot catch up by combating them with anti-oxidants. These factors are related to age-related illness and weight as well, which again, brings us back to a discussion of how they actually work.

You will see labels in Sirtuins that start with "SIR," which represents "Silence Information Regulator" genes. They do exactly that, silence or regulate, as part of their functions. The seven sirtuins that humans work with are: SIRT1, SIRT2, SIRT3, SIRT4, SIRT 5, SIRT6 and SIRT7. Each of these types is responsible for different areas of protecting cells. They work by either stimulating or turning on certain gene expressions, or by reducing and turning off other gene expressions. This essentially means that they can influence genes to do more or less of something, most of which they are already programmed to do.

Through enzyme reactions, each of the SIRT types affect different areas of cells that are responsible for the metabolic processes that help to maintain life. This is also related to what organs and functions they will affect.

For example, the SIRT6 causes an expression of genes in humans that affect skeletal muscle, fat tissue, brain, and heart. SIRT 3 would cause an expression of genes that affect the kidneys, liver, brain and heart.

If we tie these concepts together, you can see that the Sirtuin proteins can change the expression of genes, and in the case of the Sirtfood diet we care about how sirtuins can turn off those genes that are responsible for speeding up aging and for weight management.

The other aspect to this conversation of sirtuins is the function and the power of calorie restriction on the human body. Calorie restriction is simply eating less calories. This, coupled with exercise and reducing stress is usually a combination for weight loss. Calorie restriction has also proven across much research in animals and humans to increase one's lifespan.

We can look further at the role of sirtuins with calorie restriction, and using the SIRT3 protein which has a role in metabolism and aging. Amongst all of the effects of the protein on gene expression, such as preventing cells from dying, reducing tumors from growing, etc.

The SIRT3 has high expression in those metabolically active tissues as we stated earlier, and its ability to express itself increases with caloric restriction, fasting, and exercise. On the contrary, it will express itself less when the body has a high fat, high calorie-riddled diet.

The last few highlights of sirtuins are their role in regulating telomeres and reducing inflammation which also help with staving off disease and aging.

Telomeres are sequences of proteins at the ends of chromosomes. When cells divide these get shorter. As we age they get shorter, and other stressors to the body also will contribute to this. Maintaining these longer telomeres is the key to slower aging. In addition, proper diet, along with exercise and other variables can lengthen telomeres. SIRT6 is one of the sirtuins that, if activated, can help with DNA damage, inflammation and oxidative stress. SIRT1 also helps with inflammatory response cycles that are related to many age-related diseases.

Calories restriction, as we mentioned earlier, can extend life to some degree.

Since this, as well as fasting, is a stressor, these factors will stimulate the SIRT3 proteins to kick in and protect the body from the stressors and excess free radicals. Again, the telomere length is affected as well.

To sum up, all of this information also shows that, contrary to some people's beliefs that in terms of genetics, such as "it is what it is" or "it is my fate because Uncle Joe has something…" through our own lifestyle choices, and what we are exposed to, we can influence action and changes in our genes. This is quite an empowering thought, and yet another reason why you should be excited to have a science-based diet such as the Sirtfood diet, available to you.

Having laid this all out before you, you should be able to appreciate how and why these miraculous compounds work in your favor, to keep you youthful, healthy, and lean If they are working hard for you, don't you feel that you should do something too.

Chapter 2 - Sirtfoods Basic Diet

Eating some quality foods will improve your skinny gene pathways and enables you to shed some unnecessary weight in seven days. Food such as kale, dark chocolate, and wine has a natural compounds known as polyphenols that look likes the results of fitness workout and fasting. Strawberries, cinnamon, as well as turmeric are also strong sirtfoods. These foods will activate the sirtuin steps or potential to help improve weight loss.

There Are 2 Phases To Follow The Sirtfood Diet:

Phase 1 of the Sirtfood Diet

All through the first 3 days, calorie consumption is reduced to 1,000 calories that is more than on a 5:2 fasting day. The diet involves 3 Sirtfood-full of green juices and 1 Sirtfood filled meal and 2 serves of dark chocolate.

For the remaining 4 days calories intake has to be increased to 1, 500 calories and daily day the diet should involves 2 Sirtfood-filled green juices and 2 Sirtfood-rich meals.

In the early first stage "The phase 1 stage" you are not permitted to drink any alcohol, but you are free to take water and green tea.

Phase 2 of the Sirtfood Diet

Phase 2 does not center on calorie intake reduction. Daily intake involves 3 Sirtfood-rich foods and 1 green juice, and the alternative of 1 or 2 Sirtfood crunch snacks, if necessary.

In the second phase 2 you are permitted to take red wine, but not too much they advise you to take 2-3 glasses of red wine weekly, and also water, tea, coffee and green tea.

After the Diet

You may replicate these two phases as much you desired for additional weight loss.

However, you are advised to continue Sirtifying your diet at the end of completing these phases by including sirtfoods frequently into your meals.

There are a variations of Sirtfood Diet manuals that has several recipes rich in sirtfoods. You can also add sirtfoods in your foods as a snack or in recipes you have used before. In addition, you are advised to continue taking the green juice daily.

In this manner, the Sirtfood Diet will be more of a way of lifestyle adjustment than a one-time diet.

Diet to Activate Sirtuins and Promote Health

It's apparently no accident that some of the individuals with long lifespan and healthiest populations in the world eat diets that are rich in these sirtuin activating foods, examples are those in the Mediterranean and parts of Asia. The Mediterranean diet includes polyphenol rich fruits, veggies, olive oil including red wine. The Asian diet is rich in is flavones present in soya beans and epigallactins from green tea.

Acquiring several of these health developing foods into your diet is proportionately easy. They can be included into many diets and even compound to make super-sirt meals!

Below are some grate ideas you can get started with

- Make use olive oil for frying or roasting veggies or vegetables and salad dressings.

- Ensure to own a jar of olives handy to snack on and include olives to salads or cooked meals. Tapenade usually makes a great topping for rye breads.

- Exchange usual tea and coffee for green tea. Include a press of lemon for extra interest.

- Miso alternatively can be used rather than stock cubes to flavor soups and stews. Milder light colored miso may be used as a spread. Miso soup makes a great snack or soft meal if presented with salad or bread.

- Include tofu or tempeh to stir fries. Mix silken tofu into soups, immerse and creamy desserts.

- Put berries, blackcurrants to muesli, smoothies and juices. Fresh yoghurt as well as fresh berries ensure a healthy snack or dessert.

- Take your greens. Cabbage and broccoli are outstanding support to any meal and can also be included to stir fries, curries, stews and casseroles.

- Enrich up your life with turmeric and other spices. Don't restrict your input of seasonings to curries, include them to grains and vegetables.

- Include cacao powder to smoothies and desserts too. Dredge cacao nibs on salads or include to trail mixes.

.

Sirt food meal plan is divided into 2 phases. Phase 1 includes the first three days of the plan. While phase 2 consists of the last four days of the diet plan.

Sirt Food Seven Days Plan

7 DAYS SIRTFOOD MEAL PLAN			
DAY	BREAKFAST	LUNCH	DINNER
PHASE I			
1	Green Juice	Chicken stir-fry	Green Juice
2	Berry juice	Tina salad	Berry juice
3	Green juice	Aromatic chicken breast + kale and red onions + a tomato and chili salsa	Green juice
PHASE 2			
1	Sirtfood Cereal	Green juice	Asian King Prawn Stir-Fry with Buckwheat Noodles
2	Strawberry buckwheat tabouleh	Green juice	Pita pizza

| 3 | Sirtfood bites | Berry juice | Meat loaf pita sandwich |
| 4 | Sirt Muesli | Green juice | Aromatic Chicken Breast + Kale and Red Onions + a Tomato and Chili Salsa |

Chapter 3 - Top 20 Sirtfoods

Sirtfoods are plant-based foods that activate a called a sirtuin. Sirtuins belong to a family of proteins that help insulate and protect our cells from damage, reducing our risk of developing any or all major diseases.

Many people turn to diets as a means of losing weight, and the Sirtfood Diet has been proven to be very good at helping achieve this goal. However, the interesting finding is that the diet isn't a weight management tool, so much as a strategy for enhancing overall health, in order to live longer, healthier lives, free from diabetes, heart disease, and even dementia. It simply turns out that healthy body weight is a natural by-product of good health.

Unfortunately, the Standard American Diet SAD, also sometimes referred to as the Western Pattern Diet WPD, is notably lacking in sirtfoods.

I'll introduce you to a list of the Top 20 Sirtfoods, which are featured prominently. I've also included a supplementary list of an additional 10 fruits and 10 vegetables that are also very rich in sirtuin-activators and also common throughout these recipes.

This makes the recipes not only feel somewhat familiar and achievable, but by sticking to the top sirtfoods, it makes shopping convenient and easy. You'll get to know the ingredients quickly and develop your confidence for tweaking recipes and developing your own, unique versions.

Healthy, home cooked food should never be boring or distasteful, and they don't have to be difficult either. Plants have such an incredible array of flavors and aromas that you'll find your Sirtfood meals exciting and packed with just as much flavor as nutrition.

Top 20 Sirtfoods

In Alphabetical Order:

1. Arugula Rocket
2. Buckwheat
3. Capers
4. Celery
5. Chili's
6. Cocoa
7. Coffee
8. Extra Virgin Olive Oil
9. Garlic
10. Green Tea
11. Kale
12. Medjool Dates
13. Parsley
14. Red Endive

15. Red Onions
16. Red Wine
17. Soy
18. Strawberries
19. Turmeric
20. Walnuts

Additional Sirtuin Rich Foods

Fruits

- Apples
- Blackberries
- Black currents
- Blueberries
- Citrus fruits
- Cranberries
- Goji berries
- Plums
- Raspberries
- Red Grapes

Vegetables and Herbs

- Artichokes
- Asparagus

- Broccoli

- Chia seeds

- Dill

- Green beans

- Lovage

- Quinoa

- Shallots

- Spinach

- Watercress

There are plenty of other vitamin rich and nutrient dense plants for you to add to your meals as well. Whenever you're in doubt or looking to experiment with new ingredients, simply look for the freshest, seasonal produce you can find, preferably in a wide array of colors. This combination will gift you with plenty of nutrition whether or not the individual items made the top 20 list of Sirtfoods.

As you're trying out the recipes on the following pages, don't be afraid to add or swap ingredients, especially if you know you detest certain options and can't get enough of others.

This guide is meant to last you a lifetime, so mark up the pages and add your own personal flair as you test out new dishes and become more and more addicted to the health and vitality that comes from eating a diverse, nutritional diet.

Chapter 4 - Why Choosing Sirt-food Diet/Benefits of This Diet

Sirtfoods are nearly all nutritious choices and might even cause a few health benefits due to their anti-inflammatory properties. Yet eating a small number of mainly well-balanced meals can't meet most of your system's nutrient needs. The Sirtfood diet is restrictive and will be offering no clear, exceptional health and fitness benefits over another sort of diet plan. Moreover, eating just 1000 calories is on average not recommended with no oversight of a doctor. Eating 1,500 calories a day is too restrictive for a lot of men and women.

The diet additionally requires drinking two to three green juices every day. Even though juices can become quite a very good supply of minerals and vitamins, they're also a supply of sugars and also comprise nearly none of the nutritious fiber which whole vegetables and fruits do.

What is more, sipping juice all through the entire afternoon is a terrible idea for the blood glucose along with your own teeth. Perhaps not obviously, since the diet is indeed restricted in food and calorie choice, it really is most likely deficient in protein, minerals, and vitamins, particularly throughout the first phase.

Because of the minimal-carb levels along with restrictive eating food choices, this diet might be tricky to stick to for the full 3 weeks.

In addition to the high first expenses of needing to buy a juicer, even the publication along with certain infrequent and costly ingredients, in addition to enough timing costs of organizing specific juices and meals, this particular diet becomes laborious and disheartening for lots of men and women.

Safety and Unwanted Effects

Even though the very initial phase of this Sirtfood diet is very low in carbs and incomplete, there aren't any true security concerns for the average, healthy adult considering that the diet lasts for a short time.

Yet for somebody with diabetes, metabolic limitation and drinking mainly juice for the first day or two of this diet might cause dangerous fluctuations in glucose. Nonetheless, a good wholesome person could experience some unwanted effects — mainly appetite.

Eating just 1000 - 1,500 calories every day will render only about anybody feeling hungry, particularly if much about that which you are consuming is juice that will be low in fiber, a nutritional supplement which will help keep you feeling full.

Throughout the phase, you may possibly experience other negative effects like fatigue, light-headedness, and irritability as a result of calorie limitation.

For a healthy adult, acute health consequences are improbable when the diet has been followed closely for just three weeks.

Sirtfoods Together With Additional Foods

We realize that sirtfoods plus several different foods are beneficial to all of us, whether veggies such as broccoli or berries, spices such as garlic, or beverages such as green tea. The main reason that these -- and a number of other plant foods -- are all advantageous to people, is primarily to the bio-active plant chemicals they contain. For the savvy, we're thinking about sulforaphane from broccoli, lycopene from tomatoes, cur cumin from turmeric, and catechins from green tea extract. All the focus of extensive scientific research is trying to explain why those foods are really great for our wellbeing.

However, as opposed to simply eating those foods that are individual, nearly as effective as they truly are, imagine us mixing food items – and for that reason, their nourishment – together at meals delivered a much larger health boost? Imagine if we can make synergies between nutrition in various foods that enhance their health benefits? It's a fresh concept, also below are a few types of the foods and you also may recognize the sirtfoods on this list may create optimum effect.

1. Green-tea lemon: green tea drinkers may get various health advantages given that swallowing this particular precious drink is related to less cancer, cardiovascular disease, obesity, and diabetes. All these health benefits are clarified by its own unique material of plant chemicals called catechins, and notably, a sort identified as epigallocatechin gal late. Adding a dab of lemon juice into a green tea that will be full of vitamin helps significantly raise the number of catechins that have absorbed into the human body.

2. Tomato-sauce + extra virgin coconut oil: lycopene may be your carotenoid liable for its deep crimson color of berries, and its own ingestion is connected with a reduced risk of certain cancers mainly cancer of the prostate, cardiovascular disease, obesity, and shielding the skin against the damaging effects of sunlight. The first point to learn about lycopene is that processing and cooking berries considerably advance the total amount of lycopene the human body is able to consume. The reason is the fact that the existence of fat farther increases lycopene absorption. Therefore, in your chosen dishes having a generous drizzle of extra virgin coconut oil makes sense.

3. Turmeric + black pepper: turmeric, the glowing yellow spice ever-present in traditional Indian cooking, could be the topic of intense study because of its anti-cancer properties, its own capability to decrease inflammation within the torso, also even for

staving off dementia. That is thought to be primarily as a result of the active ingredient cur cumin. However, the issue with cur cumin is it is extremely poorly absorbed by your system. But adding black pepper increases its absorption, which makes them the most ideal spice for increased benefits. Cooking garlic in liquid and fat, also further helps with cur cumin absorption.

4. Broccoli + steak: it is no secret that broccoli is very good for people, together with benefits including reducing cancer risk. Broccoli's main cancer-preventive component is sulforaphane. That really is formed once people eat broccoli by the actions of a molecule discovered in broccoli known as myrosinase. But cooking broccoli, mainly overcooking it, begins to destroy the myrosinase enzyme, reducing the total amount of sulforaphane that may be made. Actually, if we aren't careful, we may cook the advantages directly from broccoli. But for people that enjoy their carrot well-cooked in the place of gently cooked for two to four minutes, adding in additional all-natural origins of myrosinase, like out of mustard or horseradish, implies that sulforaphane may still be produced.

5. Salad + avocado: green leafy veggies like spinach, spinach, and watercress, are packed filled with health-promoting carotenoids like immune-strengthening beta-carotene along with eye-friendly lutein. But when eaten raw, in the kind of sausage, those carotenoids are somewhat more challenging to consume. However, the accession of a few fats can truly help with this and

adding avocado, full of fat, into some salad proved to radically boost the number of carotenoids that can be consumed.

25

Chapter 5 - Recommended Recipes

Breakfast

1. Creamy Strawberry & Cherry Smoothie

- Preparation Time: 10 minutes
- Cooking Time: 15 minutes
- Servings: 1

Ingredients:

- 100g 3½ oz. strawberries
- 75g 3oz frozen pitted cherries
- 1 tablespoon plain full-fat yogurt
- 175mls 6fl oz. unsweetened soya milk

Directions:

Place the ingredients into a blender then process until smooth. Serve and enjoy.

Nutrition:

132 calories per serving

2. Strawberry & Citrus Blend

- Preparation Time: 10 minutes
- Cooking Time: 15 minutes
- Servings: 1

Ingredients:

- 75g 3oz strawberries
- 1 apple, cored
- 1 orange, peeled
- ½ avocado, peeled and de-stoned
- ½ teaspoon matcha powder
- Juice of 1 lime

Directions:

Place ingredients into a blender with enough water to cover them and process until smooth.

Nutrition:

272 calories per serving

3. Grapefruit & Celery Blast

- Preparation Time: 10 minutes
- Cooking Time: 15 minutes

- Servings: 1

Ingredients

- 1 grapefruit, peeled
- 2 stalks of celery
- 50g 2oz kale
- ½ teaspoon matcha powder

Directions:

Place ingredients into a blender with water to cover them and blitz until smooth.

Nutrition:

71 calories per serving

4. Orange & Celery Crush

- Preparation Time: 10 minutes
- Cooking Time: 15 minutes
- Servings: 1

Ingredients:

- 1 carrot, peeled
- 3 stalks of celery
- 1 orange, peeled

- ½ teaspoon matcha powder

- Juice of 1 lime

Directions:

Place ingredients into a blender with enough water to cover them and blitz until smooth.

Nutrition:

95 calories per serving

5. Tropical Chocolate Delight

- Preparation Time: 10 minutes

- Cooking Time: 15 minutes

- Servings: 1

Ingredients

- 1 mango, peeled & de-stoned

- 75g 3oz fresh pineapple, chopped

- 50g 2oz kale

- 25g 1oz rocket

- 1 tablespoon 100% cocoa powder or cacao nibs

- 150mls 5fl oz. coconut milk

Direction

Place ingredients into a blender and blitz until smooth. You can add a little water if it seems too thick.

Nutrition:

427 calories per serving

6. Walnut & Spiced Apple Tonic

- Preparation Time: 10 minutes
- Cooking Time: 15 minutes
- Servings: 1

Ingredients

- 6 walnuts halves
- 1 apple, cored
- 1 banana
- ½ teaspoon matcha powder
- ½ teaspoon cinnamon
- Pinch of ground nutmeg

Directions:

Place ingredients into a blender and add sufficient water to cover them. Blitz until smooth and creamy.

Nutrition:

95 calories per serving

Main Meals

7. Coq Au Vin

- Preparation Time: 10 minutes
- Cooking Time: 15 minutes
- Servings: 8

Ingredients:

- 450g 1lb button mushrooms
- 100g 3½oz streaky bacon, chopped
- 16 chicken thighs, skin removed
- 3 cloves of garlic, crushed
- 3 tablespoons fresh parsley, chopped
- 3 carrots, chopped
- 2 red onions, chopped
- 2 tablespoons plain flour
- 2 tablespoons olive oil
- 750mls 1¼ pints red wine
- 1 bouquet grain

Directions:

In a large plate, put the flour and coat the chicken in it. Heat the olive oil then add the chicken and brown it, before setting aside. Fry the bacon in the pan then add the onion and cook for 5 minutes. Pour in the red wine and add the chicken, carrots, bouquet grain and garlic. Transfer it to a large ovenproof dish. Cook at 180C/360F for an hour. Remove the bouquet grain and skim off any excess fat, if necessary. Add in the mushrooms and cook for 15 minutes. Stir in the parsley just before serving.

Nutrition:

459 calories per serving

8. Turkey Satay Skewers

- Preparation Time: 10 minutes
- Cooking Time: 15 minutes
- Servings: 2

Ingredients

- 250g 9oz turkey breast, cubed
- 25g 1oz smooth peanut butter
- 1 clove of garlic, crushed
- ½ small bird's eye chili or more if you like it hotter, finely

chopped

- ½ teaspoon ground turmeric
- 200mls 7fl oz. coconut milk
- 2 teaspoons soy sauce

Directions:

Combine the coconut milk, peanut butter, turmeric, soy sauce, garlic and chili. Add the turkey pieces to the bowl and stir them until they are completely coated. Push the turkey onto metal skewers. Place the satay skewers on a barbeque or under a hot grill broiler and cook for 4-5 minutes on each side, until they are completely cooked.

Nutrition:

431 calories per serving

9. Salmon & Capers

- Preparation Time: 10 minutes
- Cooking Time: 15 minutes
- Servings: 4

Ingredients

- 75g 3oz Greek yogurt
- 4 salmon fillets, skin removed

- 4 teaspoons Dijon Mustard
- 1 tablespoon capers, chopped
- 2 teaspoons fresh parsley
- Zest of 1 lemon

Directions:

Put the yogurt, mustard, lemon zest, parsley and capers in a mixing bowl. Thoroughly coat the salmon in the mixture. Place the salmon under a hot grill broiler and cook for 3-4 minutes on each side, or until the fish is cooked. Serve with mashed potatoes and vegetables or a large green leafy salad.

Nutrition:

321 calories per serving

10. Moroccan Chicken Casserole

- Preparation Time: 10 minutes
- Cooking Time: 15 minutes
- Servings: 4

Ingredients

- 250g 9oz tinned chickpeas garbanzo beans drained
- 4 chicken breasts, cubed
- 4 Medrol dates, halved

- 6 dried apricots, halved
- 1 red onion, sliced
- 1 carrot, chopped
- 1 teaspoon ground cumin
- 1 teaspoon ground cinnamon
- 1 teaspoon ground turmeric
- 1 bird's-eye chili, chopped
- 600mls 1 pints chicken stock broth
- 25g 1oz corn flour
- 60mls 2fl oz. water
- 2 tablespoons fresh coriander

Directions:

Place the chicken, chickpeas garbanzo beans, onion, carrot, chili, cumin, turmeric, cinnamon and stock broth into a large saucepan. Put it to the boil, and reduce heat after that simmer for 25 minutes. Add in the dates and apricots and simmer for 10 minutes. In a cup, mix the corn flour together with the water until it becomes a smooth paste. Pour the mixture into the saucepan and stir until it thickens. Add in the coriander cilantro and mix well. Serve with buckwheat or couscous.

Nutrition:

401 calories per serving

11. Chili Con Carne

- Preparation Time: 10 minutes
- Cooking Time: 15 minutes
- Servings: 4

Ingredients

- 450g 1lb lean minced beef
- 400g 14oz chopped tomatoes
- 200g 7oz red kidney beans
- 2 tablespoons tomato purée
- 2 cloves of garlic, crushed
- 2 red onions, chopped
- 2 bird's-eye chilies, finely chopped
- 1 red pepper bell pepper, chopped
- 1 stick of celery, finely chopped
- 1 tablespoon cumin
- 1 tablespoon turmeric
- 1 tablespoon cocoa powder
- 400mls 14 FL oz. beef stock broth
- 175mls 6fl oz. red wine
- 1 tablespoon olive oil

Directions:

Put the oil in a saucepan then add the onion and cook for 5 minutes. Add in the garlic, celery, chili, turmeric, and cumin and cook for 2 minutes before adding then meat then cook for another 5 minutes. Pour in the stock broth, red wine, tomatoes, tomato purée, red pepper bell pepper, kidney beans and cocoa powder. Let it simmer for 45 minutes, keep it covered and stirring occasionally. Serve with brown rice or buckwheat.

Nutrition:

390 calories per serving

12. Prawn & Coconut Curry

- Preparation Time: 10 minutes
- Cooking Time: 15 minutes
- Servings: 4

Ingredients

- 400g 14oz tinned chopped tomatoes
- 400g 14oz large prawns shrimps, shelled and raw
- 25g 1oz fresh coriander cilantro chopped
- 3 red onions, finely chopped
- 3 cloves of garlic, crushed
- 2 bird's eye chilies
- ½ teaspoon ground coriander cilantro
- ½ teaspoon turmeric
- 400mls 14fl oz. coconut milk

- 1 tablespoons olive oil
- Juice of 1 lime

Directions:

Place the onions, garlic, tomatoes, chilies, lime juice, turmeric, ground coriander, chilies and half of the fresh coriander cilantro into a blender and blitz until you have a smooth curry paste. In a frying pan, put the oil, add the paste and cook for 2 minutes. Stir in the coconut milk and warm it thoroughly. Add the prawn's shrimps to the paste and cook them until they have turned pink and are completely cooked. Stir in the fresh coriander cilantro. Serve with rice.

Nutrition:

322 calories per serving

Desserts

13. Choc Nut Truffles

- Preparation Time: 10 minutes
- Cooking Time: 15 minutes
- Servings: 1

Ingredients

- 150g 5oz desiccated shredded coconut

- 50g 2oz walnuts, chopped
- 25g 1oz hazelnuts, chopped
- 4 Medrol dates
- 2 tablespoons 100% cocoa powder or cacao nibs
- 1 tablespoon coconut oil

Directions:

Place ingredients into a blender and process until smooth and creamy. Using a teaspoon, scoop the mixture into bite-size pieces then roll it into balls. Place them into small paper cases, cover them and chill for 1 hour before serving.

Nutrition:

236 calories per serving

14. No-Bake Strawberry Flapjacks

- Preparation Time: 10 minutes
- Cooking Time: 15 minutes
- Servings: 1

Ingredients

- 75g 3oz porridge oats
- 125g 4oz dates
- 50g 2oz strawberries

- 50g 2oz peanuts unsalted
- 50g 2oz walnuts
- 1 tablespoon coconut oil
- 2 tablespoons 100% cocoa powder or cacao nibs

Directions:

Place ingredients into a blender and process until they become a soft consistency. Spread the mixture onto a baking sheet or small flat tin. Press the mixture down and smooth it out. Cut it into 8 pieces, ready to serve. You can add an extra sprinkling of cocoa powder to garnish if you wish.

Nutrition:

182 calories each

15. Chocolate Balls

- Preparation Time: 10 minutes
- Cooking Time: 15 minutes
- Servings: 1

Ingredients

- 50g 2oz peanut butter or almond butter
- 25g 1oz cocoa powder
- 25g 1oz desiccated shredded coconut

- 1 tablespoon honey
- 1 tablespoon cocoa powder for coating

Directions:

Mix all ingredients into a bowl. Scoop out a little of the mixture and shape it into a ball. Roll the ball in a little cocoa powder and set aside. Repeat for the remaining mixture. Can be eaten straight away or stored in the fridge.

Nutrition:

115 calories per serving

16. Warm Berries & Cream

- Preparation Time: 10 minutes
- Cooking Time: 15 minutes
- Servings: 1

Ingredients:

- 250g 9oz blueberries
- 250g 9oz strawberries
- 100g 3½ oz. redcurrants
- 100g 3½ oz. blackberries
- 4 tablespoons fresh whipped cream
- 1 tablespoon honey

Directions:

Mix all ingredients into a bowl. Scoop out a little of the mixture and shape it into a ball. Roll the ball in a little cocoa powder and set aside. Repeat for the remaining mixture. Can be eaten straight away or stored in the fridge.

Nutrition:

115 calories per serving

17. Zest and Juice of 1 Orange

- Preparation Time: 10 minutes
- Cooking Time: 15 minutes
- Servings: 4

Ingredients:

- 250g 9oz blueberries
- 1 tablespoon honey
- Juice of 1 orange
- 4 tablespoons fresh whipped cream

Directions:

Place all of the berries into a pan along with the honey and orange juice. Gently heat the berries for around 5 minutes until warmed through. Serve the berries into bowls and add a dollop of whipped cream on top. Alternatively you could top them off with from age frays or yogurt.

Nutrition:

180 calories per serving

18. Chocolate Fondue

- Preparation Time: 10 minutes
- Cooking Time: 15 minutes
- Servings: 1

Ingredients:

- 125g 4oz dark chocolate min 85% cocoa
- 300g 11oz strawberries
- 200g 7oz cherries
- 2 apples, peeled, cored and sliced
- 100mls 3½ FL oz. double cream heavy cream

Directions:

In a fondue pot or saucepan, place the chocolate and cream then warm it until smooth and creamy. Serve in the fondue pot or transfer it to a serving bowl. Scatter the fruit on a serving dish ready to be dipped into the chocolate.

Nutrition:

352 calories per serving

19. Walnut & Date Loaf

- Preparation Time: 10 minutes
- Cooking Time: 15 minutes
- Servings: 12

Ingredients

- 250g 9oz self-rising flour
- 125g 4oz Medrol dates, chopped
- 50g 2oz walnuts, chopped
- 250mls 8fl oz. milk
- 3 eggs
- 1 medium banana, mashed
- 1 teaspoon baking soda

Directions:

Sieve the baking soda and flour into a bowl. Add in the banana, eggs, milk and dates and combine all the ingredients thoroughly. Transfer the mixture to a lined loaf tin and smooth it out. Scatter the walnuts on top. Bake the loaf in the oven at 180C/360F for 45 minutes. Serve!

Nutrition:

166 calories per serving

20. Strawberry Frozen Yogurt

- Preparation Time: 10 minutes
- Cooking Time: 15 minutes
- Servings: 4

Ingredients

- 450g 1lb plain yogurt
- 175g 6oz strawberries
- Juice of 1 orange
- 1 tablespoon honey

Directions:

Place the strawberries and orange juice into a food processor or blender and blitz until smooth. Press the mixture through a sieve into a large bowl to remove seeds. Stir in the honey and yogurt. Transfer the mixture to an ice-cream maker and follow the manufacturer's instructions. Alternatively pour the mixture into a container and place in the fridge for 1 hour. Use a fork to whisk it and break up ice crystals and freeze for 2 hours.

Nutrition:

133 calories per serving

Chapter 6 - How Much Sirtfood Do You Need To Eat?

Any diet that professes to turn on your "thin qualities" makes certain to knock some people's socks off—and undoubtedly set off your B.S. locator. However, that is actually what the Sirtfood Diet professes to do.

This diet, which hit the scene in 2016, encountered a flood in fame when news broke that Adele, Pippa Middleton, and different big names purportedly follow the arrangement to get thinner and lift vitality with nourishments like kale, red wine, dim chocolate, and matcha—and it's just been picking up steam. Truth be told, Google recently declared that the Sirtfood Diet was the seventh-most looked for diet in 2019.

In any case, how precisely is this diet arranged, and what's a "Sirtfood," in any case? Spoiler: This arrangement might be stacked with supplements, yet a few specialists state it's not so much dependent on strong science. This is what you have to know.

The Sirtfood Diet was created by U.K. - based nutritionists Aidan Goggins and Glen Matten, both of whom hold graduate degrees in nourishing medication. The Sirtfood Diet, was distributed in the U.S. in 2017 and highlights an arrangement to enable you "to shed seven pounds in seven days while encountering enduring vitality and getting a charge out of the nourishments you love including chocolate, red wine, strawberries, and then some."

The reason of the Sirtfood Diet.

The fundamental reason of the Sirtfood Diet is that sure nourishments, named sirtfoods, can basically imitate the demonstrated advantages of caloric limitation and fasting by method for actuating Sirtuins proteins in the body extending from SIRT1 to SIRT7 that control natural pathways, turn certain qualities on and off, and help shield cells from age-related decay. Actuation of SIRT1, for instance, has been appeared in some lab and creature concentrates to instigate the development of new mitochondria, expand life range, and improve oxidative digestion, which may bolster weight loss and support.

Since fasting and extreme caloric limitation is extremely hard and often, not fitting, Goggins and Matten built up their dietary arrangement—concentrated on eating heaps of "sirtfoods"— as a simpler method to animate the body's sirtuin qualities in some cases alluded to as "thin qualities" and in this manner increase weight loss and advance by and large wellbeing.

What makes something a "Sirtfood"?

Some "Sirtfoods" that Goggins and Matten incorporate green tea, berries, cocoa powder, turmeric, kale, onions, parsley, arugula, chilies, espresso, red wine, pecans, escapades, buckwheat, and olive oil. These nourishments contain specific polyphenol mixes quercetin, resveratrol, kaempferol, and so forth. That have, truth be told, been found in scientific examinations to increment sirtuin movement. Thus, in such manner, the diet is in any event to some degree dependent on science.

The issue, notwithstanding, is that these nourishments may not contain adequate degrees of these polyphenols to really initiate sirtuins in any important manner. A considerable lot of the examinations connecting polyphenol mixes to expanded sirtuin movement have just been done on profoundly thought types of these mixes.

How The Sirtfood Diet Is Organized.

The Sirtfood Diet is separated into two fundamental stages.

Stage one goes on for seven days. For the initial three days, the diet calls for expending three Sirtfood green juices and one feast rich in sirtfoods for a sum of 1,000 calories for every day. Days four through seven each comprise of two green juices and two dinners for an aggregate of 1,500 calories for every day. This is the piece of the arrangement wherein Goggins and Matten guarantee you can "shed seven pounds in seven days."

Stage Two is a 14-day support stage intended to "assist you with getting more fit consistently." You can have three Sirtfood-rich dinners in addition to one green juice for every day.

As per Goggins and Matten, these two stages can be rehashed as often as you'd like for a weight loss help. Following these underlying three weeks, you're urged to keep certifying your dinners by eating a rich in sirtfoods diet staying aware of your everyday green juice.

What do practical sustenance specialists need to state about it?

Generally speaking, master criticism on the Sirtfood Diet is blended. The uplifting news: The diet seems to be stacked with nourishments that are solid. "There is broad research that features the numerous advantages of a portion of the nourishments got down on about this diet, similar to espresso, green tea, dim chocolate, and dull verdant greens," says Jessica Cording, R.D., enrolled dietitian and wellbeing mentor.

Huge numbers of these nourishments may likewise bolster sound weight loss, says Frances Largeman-Roth, R.D., yet whether they advance weight loss by actuating sirtuins stays to be demonstrated. As indicated by Largeman-Roth, while considers have demonstrated the significance of sirtuins and sirtuin-boosting mixes on metabolic pathways, there is no science behind the capacity of specific nourishments to help sirtuin levels.

"The nourishments advanced on the diet are ones that battle irritation and would be valuable for anybody to add to their diet yet not on the grounds that they help sirtuins," she says. "Because a nourishment contains a specific supplement connected to digestion doesn't imply that nourishment causes programmed weight loss—it is highly unlikely to turn on a 'thin quality' with nourishment."

Furthermore, while these "sirtfoods" are undoubtedly solid, Largeman-Roth says somebody would need to ensure they're likewise balancing their dinners with sound fats and proteins.

With respect to the structure of the diet, it may not be great, however it could be a receptive choice for individuals who are keen on a weight loss plan that has some structure and offers space for adaptability and customization. "I welcome that it's a 'diet of consideration' versus one concentrated essentially on limiting nourishments," she says.

All things considered, Cording concedes that the juice-substantial starting piece of Phase One is a piece lower in calories than what she'd normally suggest, however in the late stages, which incorporate an unhealthier objective and strong nourishment, are to some degree increasingly feasible.

Proceed, eat more "sirtfoods," however perhaps reconsider before really focusing on the Sirtfood Diet. Both Cording and Largeman-Roth concur that plant-based, cell reinforcement pressed "sirtfoods" can make an effectively solid expansion to your diet and assist support with weighting loss or sound weight upkeep.

Any weight loss from following a Sirtfood Diet could almost certainly be credited to eating less calories, more fiber, and devouring more supplements when all is said in done—which you could involvement in any number of dietary methodologies. If you would like to attempt it, ensure you remember to incorporate a lot of solid fats and protein a Mediterranean-style diet supported with extra "sirtfoods" would be a decent spot to begin, and consider counseling with an enlisted dietitian for help altering an arrangement that is custom fitted for your specific needs and objectives.

It's just every so often that a diet goes along that changes the manner in which we consider nourishment. The last one, was most likely 5:2, the fasting diet.

Presently, comes the Sirtfood diet. It's radical since it rethinks what a few nourishments accomplish for us, reclassifies the idea of a super food – and will make you need to eat certain food sources each day, for the remainder of your life.

"The Sirtfood diet unites the most advantageous nourishments on earth into a progressive better approach for eating," as indicated by sustenance specialists Aiden Goggins and Glen Matten. These nourishments - which they've named Sirtfoods - have, they state been appeared to actuate fat consuming yet in addition advance muscle development, support and fix.

Beneath, the creators clarify why eating Sirtfoods is such a progressive dietary methodology:

What are Sirtfoods and for what reason would they say they are so unique?

Sirtfoods are a newfound gathering of nourishments that turn on a ground-breaking reusing process in the body that gets out cell waste and consumes fat. They do this by initiating our sirtuin 'thin' qualities – similar qualities enacted by exercise and fasting.

Alongside fat consuming, Sirtfoods likewise have the extraordinary capacity to normally satisfy craving and increment muscle work. It is settled that the way of life eating the most Sirtfoods have been the least fatty and most advantageous on the planet. What does the Sirtfood Diet involve?

Stage 1 of the Sirtfood Diet is the hyper-achievement stage, a 7-day plan demonstrated to help lose 7lbs. During the initial three days, calorie admission is limited to 1,000 calories for every day, comprising of three Sirtfood green juices, in addition to one full dinner rich in Sirtfoods. On day's four to seven, calorie admission increments to 1,500 calories, containing two Sirtfood-rich green juices and two Sirtfood-rich suppers.

Stage 2 is a 14-day support stage, where weight loss proceeds relentlessly. This is accomplished by eating three adjusted Sirtfood-rich suppers day by day, alongside a 'support' Sirtfood green juice.

Is the diet feasible over an extensive stretch of time?

We realize that the main effective diets over the long haul are diets of incorporation, not avoidance. In light of that rule, something we love is the possibility of 'sirtifying' your suppers, with stacks more goodness on account of some basic swaps and Sirtfood incorporations.

Chapter 7 - Sirtfood Diet Tips

Unlike fasting, the Sirtfood diet doesn't involve skipping meals in order to experience the benefits it can offer. Therefore, you are not going through starvation to reach your weight loss and health goals. The diet involves calorie restriction meaning, you lower the number of calories you consume on a daily basis, but you will still have breakfast, lunch, dinner, and even desserts or snacks. Now you are probably wondering, "How am I going to lose pounds by eating three meals a day?" The secret lies within the meal plan, as it can seriously deliver amazing results.

The founders of the diet promise that you will lose seven pounds in the first seven days. This may sound too good to be true, but it is clinically proven. Not all bodies react the same to this diet, so the weight loss can be more or less visible. This diet promises to deliver, so you will have outstanding results for trying it. Since you will feel a lot more energized compared to your normal diet, why not put the excess energy to good use? Plenty of athletes from the UK have tried this diet, so you can easily conclude that it works perfectly fine with training and workout. In order to maximize the fat-burning effect, I would highly recommend workouts, but it is up to you how intense you want to train.

When you are satisfied with the weight you lost so far, you can simply go into the maintenance phase of this diet. Sounds neat, right? This is what's great about this diet — it gives you the possibility to preserve your weight, unlike many other radical diets. Most people following a diet complain that they start to gain weight immediately after quitting the diet. These radical diets don't have a preservation mode, so they don't give you the chance to enjoy the weight you lost.

This diet has some major advantages compared to other meal plans or programs designed to lose weight and get healthier. The ingredients are very familiar, and you can easily combine them with other foods that are not rich in sirtuins.

Also, this diet is very permissive. You can try plenty of food out there, and you are not too limited to veggies and fruits. If you are used to eating a lot, then you might think of compensating when eating these foods just to get you satisfied. There might be people trying sirtfoods and not losing weight. In this case, their problem lies within the form, variety, and quantity. It is very hard to have a meal consisting only of sirtfoods I'm referring to main meals, not snacks or desserts, so you need to find the right balance between sirtfoods and normal food. Having regular meals is very important because if you don't have the meals within a set timeframe, the diet might not work. The general rule about not eating too much at dinner or having dinner late in the evening applies.

Let's try to understand the secret of these sirtfoods. What exactly do they contain that activates sirtuins? Arugula contains nutrients like kaempferol and quercetin, capable of activating sirtuins. Buckwheat contains rutting. Capers have the same nutrients as arugula. Celery has luteolin and apigenin. Cocoa contains epicatechin. Chilies have a higher concentration of myricetin and luteolin. Coffee contains caffeic acid. Widely used in the Mediterranean diet, the extra-virgin olive oil has hydroxytyrosol and oleuropein. Kale contains the same nutrients as arugula and capers. You can find ajoene and myricetin in garlic. In green tea, you can find EGCG epigallocatechin gallate. Medjool dates contain caffeic and Gallic acid. Parsley has myricetin and apigenin. In red endives, you can find luteolin. Quercetin can be found in red onions. Strawberries contain fisetin. Walnuts are a great source of Gallic acid. Turmeric has cur cumin. Soy contains formononetin and daidzein. Red wine has piceatannol and resveratrol.

Now you are probably wondering why I'm bothering you with these fancy names of nutrients. Indeed, they all have the power to trigger sirtuins, but as it turns out, our standard diet is very poor when it comes to these nutrients. Researchers have proven that a standard US diet only contains 13 milligrams daily value of five key sirtuin-activating nutrients apigenin, luteolin, kaempferol, myricetin, and quercetin. In Japan, daily intake is five times higher. Well, a proper Sirtfood diet should allow you to consume hundreds of milligrams of these important ingredients per day. Obviously, if you manage to introduce most of the ingredients and sirtfoods mentioned above into your daily meal plan, you can effectively reap the benefits of this diet.

The nutrients mentioned above should be consumed in a natural state. This is how this diet works. You may not have the same effects if you take supplements, as the body absorbs and assimilates them a lot better in their natural form. If you take, for instance, resveratrol, this nutrient is poorly absorbed in a supplement form. However, if you consume it in a natural form, the absorption is six times higher. This should now encourage you to drink a lot of red wine. A glass of it should be more than enough. But when it comes to drinks, you need to have coffee and green tea on a daily basis. You don't have to replace water with green tea, but it is very good to have green tea a few times per day.

It is good to have as many of these sirtfoods as possible to make sure you are getting the necessary intake of sirtuin-activating nutrients. Most of them are very common or familiar, and this is the beauty of the Sirtfood diet. Therefore, it is not something extraordinary to eat garlic or red onion, strawberries, blueberries, or walnuts. It is highly recommended to make sure you include turmeric in your diet, as well.

When it comes to consuming fruits and veggies, most nutritionists would agree that it is best to consume them fresh and raw.

Eat them directly. This is how you will get all the nutrients and vitamins from them, and you will not lose anything. However, when it comes to leafy greens, it is better to juice them, as this procedure removes the low-nutrient fiber from them and allows you to have a super concentrated dose of sirtuin-activating polyphenols.

We have talked about the form and variety of the sirtfoods. Another important fact when it comes to this diet is the schedule of your meals. The Sirtfood diet should fit exactly in your busy schedule, but you need to remember to eat as early as possible in the morning.

Since this diet allows you to eat plenty of foods, it rocks when it comes to diversity. This is why you can simply feel free to consume meat, fish, and seafood if you want. As a general rule of thumb, consume less red meat beef and pork and more poultry, fish, and seafood.

The Sirtfood diet should slowly become your default meal plan. Therefore, you don't have to stick just to the four-week meal plan. Sirtuins need to be in your diet every day of the week, so why stop after finishing the fourth week? If you have a good thing running, you really don't need to interrupt it. Plus, the longer you are following this diet, the more health benefits you will experience. Sounds great, right? This should be the ultimate motivation to make you try the Sirtfood diet on a regular basis. You need to check yourself whether or not you want to prevent or even reverse some of the most common diseases caused by poor diet, slow down your aging process, and lose some weight while doing it. If it's a yes, then you need to try this diet now!

Chapter 8 - Sirtfood Science

Sirtuins & Muscle Mass

We have mentioned how sirtuins help the body retain muscle mass even when dieting. How do this work? Well, sirtuins are a group of proteins with different effects. Sirt-1 is the protein responsible for causing the body to burn fat rather than muscle for energy, which is obviously a miracle for weight loss. Another useful aspect of Sirt-1 is its ability to improve skeletal muscle.

Skeletal muscle is all the muscles you voluntarily control, such as the muscles in your limbs, back, shoulders and so on. There are two other types, cardiac muscle is what the heart is formed of, whilst smooth muscle is your involuntary muscles – which includes muscles around your blood vessels, face and various parts of organs and other tissues.

Skeletal muscle is separated into two different groups, the blandly named type-1 and type-2. Type 1 muscle is effective at continued, sustained activity whereas type-2 muscle is effective at short, intense periods of activity. So, for example, you would predominantly use type-1 muscles for jogging, but type-2 muscles for sprinting.

Sirt-1 protects the type-1 muscles, but not the type-2 muscle, which is still broken down for energy. Therefore, holistic muscle mass drops when fasting, even though type-1 skeletal muscle mass increases.

Sirt-1 also influences how the muscles actually work. Sirt-1 is produced by the muscle cells, but the ability to produce Sirt-1 decreases as the muscle ages. As a result, muscle is harder to build as you age and doesn't grow as fast in response to exercise. A lack of sirt-1 also causes the muscles to become tired quicker and gradually decline over time.

When you start to consider these effects of Sirt-1, you can start to form a picture about why fasting helps keep the body supple. Fasting releases Sirt-1, which in turn helps skeletal muscle grow and stay in good shape. Sirt-1 is also released by consuming sirtuin activators, giving the Sirtfood diet its muscle retaining power.

Sirtuins & Disease

The authors of the Sirtfood diet don't just claim that sirtuins can help improve skeletal muscle retention during dieting, but rather that they positively impact almost every dietary based disease in existence.

For example, one claim is that sirtuins help improve overall heart health by protecting and strengthening the cardiac.

Another claim expounded is that the Sirtfood diet also helps control diabetes. Some studies have found an association between Sirt-1 and the volume of insulin that can be released into the body. If you are familiar with the science behind diabetes, you may be aware that insulin is the hormone primarily responsible for controlling the levels of sugar in the blood. Therefore by increasing the amount of insulin that can be released, sirt-1 can theoretically help tackle diabetes by causing higher amounts of blood sugar to be converted into fat.

On top of this, sirtuins have been argued to influence Alzheimer's. Individuals with Alzheimer's have been found to have notably lower levels of sirtuins than healthy peers, although the mechanism of action between sirtuin and the disease is not fully understood.

The authors of the Sirtfood diet claims that sirtuins help prevent a build-up of the molecules amyloid-B and tau protein, which is responsible for the plaques that form in the brains of Alzheimer's sufferers and therefore all the corresponding symptoms. In fact, it isn't just argued that sirtuins help Alzheimer's, but also improves overall brain and cognitive function in regular people.

To add to the list of purported benefits is that sirtuins also help protect our bones. In particular, the specific argument is that sirtuin activation protects and helps retain our precious osteoblasts, which are a cell in our bones that allows more bone cells to be produced.

Finally, sirtuins have also been claimed to be a generic fighter against cancer, as they have supposedly have tumor suppression properties.

With all these claims, it is hard to discern fact from fiction. It does seem likely that a diet high in sirtuins does indeed have some of these benefits, but typically a diet high in sirtuins is more nutritious than an average Western diet. Therefore it is not yet determined whether sirtuins are the active component producing these effects, or different molecules also present in sirtfoods are responsible.

Sirtuins & Fat

Biology is far from straight-forward. You don't only have more than one type of muscle – you have more than one type of fat too. For our purposes, we are only going to focus on white adipose tissue and brown adipose tissue – two fancy terms for different kinds of fat.

White adipose tissue, or WAT as it is commonly abbreviated, is the fat made for storage. It's where your spare energy goes and having more WAT makes it easier to store and gain fat in future. Brown adipose tissue, or BAT, is a type of fat tissue that is typically associated with burning fat. BAT helps keeps us warm and contains high levels of mitochondria – the portion of the cell that is responsible for producing energy.

Leaner people actually have higher levels of brown fat than their overweight peers. BAT is located around the neck and back, whilst your WAT is located in the areas typically associated with obesity – your gut, buttocks, chest, hips. By having higher levels of BAT, fitter people have more ability to shake off calories through exercise and thermal release, so although research on BAT is still in its nascent stages, higher BAT levels and activity is hypothesized to be a good thing.

Of course, as you might now anticipate, sirtuins also affect our WAT and BAT levels. More precisely, sirtuins help convert your WAT into BAT, changing your body and making it easier to burn calories and lose weight. Over time this will produce large differences in your body composition, helping to not only make you lose weight, but become lean and fit.

Sirtfoods & Your Diet

By now, we have talked about how sirtuins are proteins produced by genes in our body, which demonstrate numerous beneficial effects on the body. We all have noted three primary means of causing sirtuins to be released in the body; eating to a calorie deficit, stringent fasting and exercise.

One of the primary claims of the Sirtfood diet is that sirtuins can also be released through your diet, with the most potent sirtuin-releasing foods nicknamed Sirtfoods. Let us examine this claim in more detail.

It is known that a nutritionally rich diet, especially a diet high in fruit and vegetables, drastically reduces the risk of cancer and a legion of diseases. The reason why this is true has been attributed to many different factors, such as the increasingly popular 'anti-oxidants' as well as higher levels of mineral and vitamins in these foods.

Yet this isn't the rationale of why the Sirtfood diet advocates so many plants and vegetables. Instead the argument rests upon Sirtfoods being special, above and beyond all other components of our food. This argument actually rests upon the toxic qualities of the Sirtfoods, rather than their nutritional superiority.

Now, this is perhaps the most fascinating aspect of the Sirtfood diet. The two authors of this diet argue that all the things we associate with improving our health exercise, fasting, and calorie restriction all have a minor stress component. Essentially these activities put the body into a minor state of stress, causing the body to enact processes that help us adapt and improve.

This concept is called hormesis and is basically the idea of what doesn't kill you, makes you stronger. Or in more scientific terms, small doses of certain harmful substances can produce a positive effect via the triggering of biological adaptations.

Plants themselves can have hormesis reactions to stressors in their environment. In fact, plant hormesis is rather sophisticated and plants, being stationary, have much more nuanced and varied stress reactions than mammals and humans.

To bring it all together, eating these hormones and chemicals from 'stressed' plants can also benefit us, as some of our biological adaptations involve usage of the same chemicals and hormones. In particular, polyphenols are known to benefit the human body and trigger sirtuin release.

This concept, of using plants stress-reactions to benefit our own is a field of study called xenohormesis. This is the very basis of Sirtfoods; sirtfoods are good for us because they contain sirtuins, which are molecules released in stress-reactions in plants, which also help our body adapt and improve.

How Much Sirtfood's Do You Need To Eat?

Of course, the Sirtfood diet is more than just pumping a bunch of the best Sirtfoods into your eating habits. It is a holistic diet with food organized into different meals, each designed to give you the highest sirtuin kick. On top of this, the Sirtfood diet isn't exotic.

The main ingredients of the Sirtfood diet are common and you probably use them already, on occasion. The trick is just making sure you are getting enough – the average American only receives 13mg of sirtuins a day – which is five times lower than their Japanese counterparts.

So if Sirtuins are so fantastic, why don't we take them as a supplement or pill? The truth is although a pharmaceutical application of sirtuins may be possible in the future our current understanding of food science and biology is still too limited for this to be effective today.

Understanding how sirtuins are processed and absorbed, which likely depends on other nutrients in food, is crucial to making sirtuins actually work. At the moment, it is simply easier and more successful to consume sirtuins the natural way, receiving all the extra stuff you need in the sirtfoods themselves.

For example, resveratrol, the sirtuin activator which is present in certain types of red wine, is known to be absorbed poorly when taken are a pure substance. When ingested in red-wine, it is in fact absorbed six times better. Simply put, food is complicated and we only understand a few pieces of the puzzle.

Another reason why sirtuins are not taken as a pill or supplement is the fact there are so many of them, all with slightly different effects. Add this to the before mentioned complexity and its better just to consume foods where you know you get a natural mix.

Chapter 9 -Fighting Fats through Sirtuins

Ecological factors significantly influence the destiny of living beings and sustenance is one of the most persuasive variables. These days life span is a significant objective of medicinal science and has consistently been a fabrication for the individual since antiquated occasions. Specifically, endeavors are planned for accomplishing effective maturing, to be specific a long life without genuine ailments, with a decent degree of physical and mental autonomy and satisfactory social connections.

Gathering information unmistakably exhibits that it is conceivable to impact the indications of maturing. Without a doubt, wholesome mediations can advance wellbeing and life span. It is commonly valued that the sort of diet can significantly impact the quality and amount of life and the Mediterranean eating regimen is paradigmatic of an advantageous dietary example

The developing cognizance of the useful impacts of a particular dietary example on wellbeing and life span in the second 50% of the only remaining century produced a ground-breaking push toward structuring eats fewer carbs that could diminish the danger of constant maladies, subsequently bringing about solid maturing. Subsequently, during the 1990s the Dietary Approaches to Stop Hypertension DASH diet was contrived so as to assess whether it was conceivable to treat hypertension not pharmacologically. To be sure, the DASH diet was very like the Mediterranean Diet, being wealthy in foods grown from the ground, entire grains, and strands, while poor in creature soaked fats and cholesterol. The awesome news leaving the investigation was that not exclusively did the DASH diet lower circulatory strain, however, it additionally diminished the danger of cardiovascular infection,

type 2 diabetes, a few sorts of malignant growth, and other maturing related maladies To additionally improve the medical advantages of plant nourishment rich, creature fat-terrible eating routines, especially in hypercholesterolemia people, the Portfolio Diet was planned This eating regimen, other than being to a great extent veggie-lover, with just limited quantities of soaked fats, prescribes likewise a high admission of utilitarian nourishments, including thick filaments, plant stanols, soy proteins, and almonds. Curiously, members on the Portfolio Diet displayed a decrease of coronary illness chance related to lower plasma cholesterol and incendiary files in contrast with members on a sound, for the most part, vegan diet.

Nonetheless, additionally, the measure of ingested nourishment has been pulling in light of a legitimate concern for mainstream researchers as a potential modifier of the harmony among wellbeing and infection in a wide range of living species. Specifically, calorie limitation CR has been exhibited to be a rising healthful intercession that animates the counter maturing instruments in the body.

In this way, the eating routine of the individuals living on the Japanese island of Okinawa has been widely broken down on the grounds that these islanders are notable for their life span and expanded wellbeing range, bringing about the best recurrence of centenarians on the planet. Interestingly, the customary Okinawan diet came about to be fundamentally the same as the Mediterranean Diet and the DASH diet regarding nourishment types. Be that as it may, the vitality admission of Okinawans, at the hour of the underlying logical perceptions, was about 20% lower than the normal vitality admission of the Japanese, along these lines deciding an average state of CR.

In his most recent examination, showing up in the Aug8 print release of the diary Cell Metabolism, he saw what happens when the SIRT1 protein is absent from fat cells, which make up muscle versus fat.

At the point when put on a high-fat eating regimen, mice coming up short on the protein began to create metabolic issues, for example, diabetes, much sooner than typical mice were given a high-fat eating routine.

"You've expelled one of the protections against metabolic decay, so on the off chance that you presently give them the trigger of a high-fat eating routine, they're considerably more delicate than the typical mouse."

The discovery raises the likelihood that medications that upgrade SIRT1 action may help ensure against weight connected illnesses. From that point forward, these proteins have been appeared to arrange an assortment of hormonal systems, administrative proteins, and different qualities, keeping cells alive and solid.

Their past work has uncovered that in the mind, SIRT1 ensures against the neurodegeneration seen in Alzheimer's, Huntington's and Parkinson's ailments.

SIRT1 is a protein that expels acetyl bunches from different proteins, changing their movement. The potential focuses of this DE acetylation are various, which is likely what gives SIRT1 its wide scope of defensive forces, Guarente says.

In the Cell Metabolism study, the specialists investigated the several qualities that were turned on in mice lacking SIRT1 yet encouraged a typical eating regimen and found that they were practically indistinguishable from those turned on in ordinary mice sustained a high-fat eating regimen.

This recommends in typical mice, improvement of the metabolic issue is a two-advance procedure. "The initial step is inactivation of SIRT1 by the high-fat eating routine, and the subsequent advance is all the terrible things that follow that," Guarente says. The scientists explored how this happens and found that in ordinary mice given a high-fat eating routine, the SIRT1 protein is cut by a compound called caspase-1, which is instigated by irritation. It's now realized that high-fat eating regimens can incite irritation, however, it's hazy precisely how that occurs, Guarente says. "What our examination says is that once you incite the fiery reaction, the outcome in the fat cells is that SIRT1 will be severed," he says.

That discovering "gives a pleasant sub-atomic system to see how fiery signals in fat tissue could prompt quick unhinging of metabolic tissue," says Anthony Suave, a partner teacher of pharmacology at Weill Cornell Medical College, who was not part of the exploration group.

Medications that focus on that incendiary procedure, just as medications that improve sirtuin action, may have some gainful remedial impact against heftiness related issues, Suave says.

Chapter 10 - The Sirtfood Diet Plan

The official Sirtfood Diet combines a short phase of calorie restriction with a long-term commitment to nutrient-dense sirtuin-activating foods.

The Difference between a Diet and Dieting

How you eat is your diet, restricting how you eat is dieting.

Aside from the first week, Stage 1, the Sirtfood diet is not a traditional diet in that, instead of simply restricting calories, you focus on increasing nutrition and improving quality.

There are only 2 stages in the Sirtfood Diet, which take up 3 weeks of your life, but those 3 weeks are designed to set the stage for incorporating sirtfoods into your lifelong diet, eliminating your need to ever resort to dieting again.

The average American over-consumes solid fats and sugars, refined grains, sodium, and saturated fat. They also under-consume vegetables, fruits, whole grains, as well as the nationally recommended intake of dairy and oils.

If this sounds like it matches your current eating patterns, don't be too hard on yourself, you're certainly not alone. And you've been practically brainwashed into adopting these poor nutrition habits.

The number of fast-food restaurants continues to grow, as do your options for pre-made, packaged foods full of empty calories and misleading promises.

When you live on a diet of these foods that are devoid of all nutrition for too long, you find yourself getting sick and overweight. So you turn to the industry that profits off of your poor health, the diet industry.

How many times have you found yourself dieting, starving yourself for weeks to lose 20 pounds? Maybe you've even been successful a time or two and lost weight, but within a few months, all the weight you lost had found its way home again, and brought a few extra friends along.

Studies show that when you restrict your calories severely for an extended period of time, you will gain the weight back as quickly as it came off, and you will do additional damage to your liver, kidneys and muscle mass as well. Short term calorie restriction, such as intermittent fasting or the first phase of the Sirtfood Diet doesn't have the same effect as depleting your body of nutrition for 3 weeks or more.

Dieting does not work.

More to the point, it's completely unnecessary, as we discovered earlier when we talked about traditional cultures and Blue Zones of the world. They don't count calories or diet, and they live to be 100+ with their full physical and mental capacities until one night, they drift off into a peaceful, joyous slumber never to wake again. That sounds a lot better than spending the last few months, if not years, of your life in a hospital bed, unable to wash or feed yourself, let alone walk around or remember your grandchildren.

You get to choose your future. And it begins with choosing a healthy diet rich in delicious, fortifying and age-defying sirtfoods.

When you're first starting to alter your diet, you may be wondering if taking supplements can help you integrate some of the sirtuin-activation benefits without the need to actually change the way you're eating. Can you just pop a pill that is full of blueberry extract or super greens?

The science is controversial on this subject but any time you're trying to cheat your way to health, chances are you will end up cheating your health instead.

If your doctor or primary care physician has advised you to take a supplement, follow their advice. There are circumstances when supplementation is critical for your survival. There are many more circumstances when taking supplements is simply advisable. Vegans, for example, are almost always deficient in vitamin B12 and Omega 3 fatty acids because both of those nutrients are most commonly found in fatty, oily fish. If following a completely plant-based diet is your ethical or moral choice, you may need to supplement for your best health.

But using supplements as a way to excuse poor dietary or lifestyle choices is never going to get you ahead in the game of life. There are many studies that suggest when certain vitamins, minerals, antioxidants or even polyphenols are isolated and consumed outside of their natural food source, they are not metabolized effectively and, in some cases, can even be detrimental to your health. Humans are very impressive in the field of science and medicine, but nature has secrets we haven't even begun to unravel, so whenever possible, it's in your best interest to find the most natural source of nutrition as possible.

Understanding Your Health Goals

You may have first heard about the Sirtfood Diet because you saw a headline about Adele's miraculous weight loss. Or perhaps you heard that scientists had discovered a "skinny gene" and the secret to accessing it was in this diet.

You want to lose weight, look great and feel great in your own skin.

That is a common and completely understandable desire, but it's not enough to get you the results you're dreaming of. At least not in the long-term. History has proven to us many times over that, even if we succeed in reaching our goal weight, either we're not satisfied or we are and we return to our old habits and the weight comes back.

One of the main reasons losing weight is ineffective is because it has an end or a result that you can achieve that allows you to give up.

If you start looking deeper and making a commitment to your health, you'll find that there is never a moment that you give yourself permission to stop. Even if you're relatively healthy today, you maintain a desire to stay healthy tomorrow, and following year, and 20 years from now. Health is a never-ending journey and that is where your true success and results will lie. You won't have a deadline to abide by and you can't fail, as long as you're taking actions every day that are designed to improve some aspect of your health.

Sometimes you'll see and feel the results right away. The participants in the first Sirtfood Diet trial saw weight loss results within 7 days. But other times, the benefits are on a cellular level and you won't realize they're making such a difference in your life until you're 80 years old and the only one of your peers that hasn't been forced to move into assisted living.

One of the other major reasons dieting has a less than impressive track record is because of the type of weight loss that is occurring.

The diseases associated with obesity aren't caused by excess weight. When you spend many years of eating unhealthy foods, you damage your metabolic system and the hormones that support your metabolism. Issues like insulin and lepton resistance cause you to gain weight and develop even more lethal diseases, like diabetes and heart disease. The food you eat is the problem, and the weight is simply a by-product of a dysfunctional metabolic system.

If you heal the system by removing the foods that are damaging your hormones and adding foods that will heal and protect your entire body, the weight will come off naturally as a result of fixing the damage.

When you try to take the weight off through calorie restriction, excessive exercise or a combination of the two, you will likely lower the numbers on your scale. There is truth to the philosophy of "calories in, calories out". However, if you aren't considering the quality of the calories going in, you won't have any control over what comes off. You're just as likely to lose water weight and muscle mass as you are to lose any fat.

If, on the other hand, you commit to providing your body with all the nutrition it needs to rebalance your hormones and protect your health, the weight that you lose is going to be the weight that you don't need: visceral fat around your vital organs and abdominal fat you've been struggling to get rid of for years. Your muscles will be protected and your body will stay nicely hydrated.

Losing weight as a result of improved health is sustainable, so it's crucial that you start to adjust your mindset and your goals if you truly want to be successful.

Summary & Key Takeaways

Your weight is not what you should be focusing on. Your health is the most important aspect of your life because, without it, you will have no joy and, most likely, very little hope of ever being able to maintain your ideal body weight.

If you prioritize health goals, you will have all the motivation you need to stop damaging your body with unhealthy foods devoid of any nutrition. You will be excited and inspired to try the myriad of fresh new ingredients that will help you feel lighter, younger, stronger and healthier than you can remember ever feeling.

The Sirtfood Diet is not about taking the easy route or popping a miracle cure pill. It's about finding the joy in your food and letting that food heal and nourish your body, allowing you to once again find joy in life. There are so many flavors waiting to be discovered, you simply need to commit to making sirtfoods the star players in your diet, with healthy proteins and fats as the phenomenal support team.

You don't have to starve yourself or even deny yourself the foods that you love, you simply have to approach food with mindfulness and awareness of the consequences it has on your body and your health.

Chapter 11 - How to Jumpstart Your Sirtfood Diet?

Being healthy and losing weight is an everyday choice. You have to take those first baby steps and see how it can change you and your life.

If you want to reap the amazing results of Sirtfoods, here is some suggested ways to jumpstart your diet:

- Safety first - Before starting any particular diet or regimen, consult your healthcare provider especially if you have an existing illnesses. This will ensure that the diet will not sabotage any medications that you might be taking or have an adverse effect to your health. Do not worry, the Sirtfood diet is fairly safe.

- Knowledge is power - This diet is still bran new, but there is still a good amount of information available and more upcoming since this diet is fast gaining popularity. In addition, you can also search the internet for recipes, food alternatives, nutrient content and more.

- Follow the guidelines - Sirtfood is guaranteed to bring results, if and only if you carefully follow the diet guide and suggested food.

- Help yourself - Aside from following what is allowed in the food program, you can start by eliminating processed and starchy food from your normal diet. Stop eating junk! This will fast track the result of Sirtfood Diet.

- Start a physical activity - Sirtfood diet can indeed burn those fats and build muscle, but I recommend that you start adding physical activities to your daily routine. A 30-minute walk a day would do wonders to your body and will also fast track the results. In addition, there are many wonderful effects when exercising like: preventing and combating health conditions, helping improve your mood, promoting better sleep, burning calories, giving you an energy boost and more.

- Hit the supermarket - The Sirtfood diet depends on certain foods. These foods were chosen because of their sirtuin-triggering ability. So if you do not follow the list, well, you won't see results. Do not worry, because I will be providing list of suggested foods; Plus there are no overly expensive type of foods and you can find it readily available almost anywhere.

- Be ready with the initial "restrictions" - Of course, if you want to see different results, you have to "sacrifice" a little in order to achieve the full benefits of the Sirtfood diet. But don't worry, the first three days are only the hardest ones for this diet since there will be calorie restrictions involved, but rest assured that it will become easier each day. Although for others who tried the diet, the restrictions set was not that hard for them, the reason is careful planning of meals. Plan your meals ahead - Whatever diet you may be on, planning your meals is a big help. Not only will it reduce the stress from dieting, you can also have the chance to weigh your choices and fill in your cupboard. For the first phase of this diet, you have to follow a calorie count. You will be surprised that there are many filling dishes allowed with less calories and packed with sirtuins.

- Involve a diet partner - This diet could also greatly benefit your family, partner or friends, plus it is easier when you have an accountability partner to remind you, share recipes with or even cook dishes with.

- Document your progress - You can start by taking "before" pictures and take necessary body measurements. You could also keep a food diary so that you can watch your food intake. Observe the changes in your body with each week or phase. You can also have a set of goals to further push you to continue with the diet.

- Be kind to yourself - Do not set too high expectations. Yes, some can easily lose 7 pounds in a week, but remember that our bodies are not all the same; and of course your level of commitment will also count. Other variables could be adding of an exercise regimen in the diet plan, which could make the losing weight process faster.

Pros and Cons of Sirtfood Diet

To help set your expectations and to further let you have a peek at the wonderful effects of the Sirtfood diet you can see the full view once you start with the diet listed below are the positive effects of the Sirtfood diet:

- All natural - Sirtfood diet promotes the consumption of all natural food. In the Sirtfood diet, most of the suggested food is plant-based. This means your body is also being detoxified from harmful chemicals, from processed food and junk food.

- Burns fat and suppress the appetite - As explained, the reason for this is that this diet taps or activates your sirtuin, as a result, fat is burned, and your appetite is suppressed. In addition, there are also food choices under Sirtfood that when consumed, can further promote burning fat since sirtuins control the genes that is in charge of your fats and sugar.

- Boosts overall health - Losing weight can definitely decrease the risk of a number of health illnesses. The food choices are all basically nutrient packed and help clean up the damage from free radicals. An example of this is green tea, with its catching component, which can fight cancer cells.

- Helps improve memory - Good news for those who are experiencing poor working memory or would like to further improve their memory, this diet is for you. Proven by studies, this diet can improve the memory depending on the food consumption. For example, consuming cocoa rich in epicatechin, another sirtuin activator and a gram of turmeric can improve the memory if they are regularly consumed.

- Acts as an antioxidant - This is mostly because the diet is rich in plant-and-fruit-based food selections, which are known to cleanse the body and get rid of the toxins.

- Helps control blood sugar - Participants of the study for this diet have shown remarkable improvements not only on the fat levels in their body, but blood sugar levels as well. This is again because of the healthy food choices. The consumption of sirtuin quercetin found in apples and onions is seen to help control the glucose levels in the body. There are more sirtuin triggers that can help regulate your sugar, imagine combining this type of food and consuming them regularly, this will definitely cause a healthier change in your body.

- Very easy to follow - Sirtfood diet is a flexible diet. There are no strict rules except to consume Sirtfoods. You can eat it on its own, add it to your regular meals or find and consume concentrated versions of suggested Sirtfood. In addition, there is no need for special supplements or pricey food types.

- No need for intense workout or starvation - Though exercise is recommended, there is no intense workout needed unless you want to try since your body is not only consuming healthier food, but is also tapping on your "skinny" gene. One thing that is guaranteed in this diet is that there is no need for fasting or starvation even during the first 3 days of the diet. You just have to make sure to plan ahead and balance your calorie intake.

- Slows the anti-ageing process - Sirtuins are actually "guardians" of the body's enzymes, which can help not only protect the cells but slows down the ageing process.

- It can fight inflammation - Due to powerful anti-oxidants present in the diet, this can help fight inflammation in the body and can help protect the heart.

- No bounce-back effect - Sirtfood diet can promote fast weight loss especially during the first week. But do not worry, during the maintenance stage, all the fat that you have shed will not return. There is no calorie-control trap in this diet. With Sirtfood diet, your tapped sirtuins actually encourages your system to burn the fat, and use the excess glucose to build the muscles, this means that fats are not stored.

In General, The Sirtfood Diet Is Safe And Effective. There Are Just A Few "Cons":

- Plateau weigh loss - This could happen in any weight loss regimen. This is a state wherein though you actively follow your weight loss program but the scale don't seem to budge. Check your food diary, level of consumption or try other sirtuin filled foods. You can also add a few minutes to your exercise time if you have any to further jumpstart your weight loss. Though this is not generally a bad thing, you just have to find the right combination of food. Be alarmed if you are suddenly gaining weight, because this means that something is wrong with your diet.

- You still have to check overall eating habits - If you're adding sirtuin-filled food to each meal but still continue to eat junk food daily or those empty calorie foods, then don't expect that the scale to bring positive results. This means that constant checking of overall consumption is still needed. Balance is the name of the game.

- Not too many materials available - Since the diet is fairly new, you may be able to find only a few resources for additional knowledge about the diet, but then there is "enough" materials, studies and testimonies to support your Sirtfood journey.

- Restrictions - Proponents of this diet assure that you will not go hungry with this food program as long as you balance your choices. But yes, the first week can be rough with the 1000/1500 restriction. But as they say, no pain, no gain! You can definitely do it.

For those who have existing medical conditions, again, please have a clearance with your health care provider before trying this diet. Note that this diet is not suitable for pregnant women who wants to maintain their weight or for women who is trying to conceive.

Before starting any diet, you should try to weigh the pros and cons. Sirtfood diet provides numerous health benefits aside from the guaranteed weight loss. For the cons, this is a matter of stepping up to the challenge and exerting the necessary effort to surpass it. Once you're fully-decided, take that first step and start with the diet!

Chapter 12 - Recipes for Sirt-food Beverages

1. Green Juice

The green juice is done mostly by weight, as it is more accurate when measuring ingredients such as leafy greens. This means you will need to have a kitchen scale on hand, which can be purchased at most grocery stores for around $10. If you can buy or grow the lavage herb, you can add in five grams for additional polyphenol benefits.

- Preparation Time: 3 minutes
- Cooking Time: 5 minutes
- Serving: 1

Ingredients:

- Kale – 75 grams
- Arugula – 30 grams
- Celery – 2 stalks
- Parsley – 5 grams
- Green apple – half
- Matcha tea powder – .5 teaspoon

Directions:

Push all of the ingredients except for the matcha and lemon through an electric juicer. Once the juicer has done its job squeeze the lemon juice into the green juice either by hand or using a hand-powered citrus juices.

Pour one-quarter of the juice into a glass, add in the matcha tea powder, and whisk until no clumps of tea remain. Stir in the remaining green juice and then drink straight away or store in the fridge for up to twenty-four hours before serving.

Nutrition:

Kilocalories per Individual 132

2. Golden Milk

This milk is full of powerful spices and soy milk to create a healthy and calming drink. You will especially find this milk helps you to sleep if you enjoy it before bed at night.

- Preparation Time: 3 minutes
- Cooking Time: 5 minutes
- Servings: 2

Ingredients:

- Soy milk, unsweetened – 3 cups

- Black pepper, ground – 1 pinch

- Ginger, ground - .25 teaspoon

- Turmeric, ground – 1.5 teaspoons

- Cinnamon stick, whole – 1

- Coconut oil – 1 tablespoon

- Date sugar – 2 tablespoons

Directions:

Stir all of the golden milk ingredients into a small saucepan and whisk to combine it over medium heat. Allow it to warm, while stirring frequently, but don't let it boil. This will take about four minutes.

Turn the heat off and taste the golden milk, adjusting it to your taste. Serve warm.

Nutrition:

Kilocalories per Individual Serving 42

3. Strawberry Apple Cider Detox Drink

Apple cider vinegar has long been shown to have many health benefits, especially when it comes to detoxing. Keep a jar of this detox drink prepared in the freezer at all times for a quick fix whenever you are feeling unwell or thirsty.

- Preparation Time: 0 minutes
- Cooking Time: 3 minutes
- Servings: 2

Ingredients:

- Water – 3 cups
- Lemon juice – 1 tablespoon
- Apple cider vinegar – 1 tablespoon
- Strawberries - .25 cup
- Honey – 1 tablespoon

Directions:

Mix all of the ingredients in a high speed blender, with or without ice, until smooth.

Divide between two serving glasses and enjoy cold.

Nutrition:

Kilocalories per Individual Serving 41

4. Cleansing Cranberry Lemon Juice Drink

Cranberries have many health benefits and are a Sirtfood. One of the many benefits is that they greatly improve your urinary tract health. Drink this juice regularly to prevent problems, or specifically when you are having symptoms that cranberries might ease.

- Preparation Time: 0 minutes
- Cooking Time: 3 minutes
- Servings 2

Ingredients:

- Cranberry juice, 100% pure and organic – 1.5 cups
- Water – 1.5 cups
- Orange juice - .25 cup
- Lemon juice – 2 tablespoons
- Honey – 2 tablespoons

Directions:

Add ingredients into a glass jar or pitcher and stir until combined. Chill in the fridge and serve cold.

Nutrition:

Kilocalories per Individual Serving 90

5. Ginger Turmeric Wellness Shots

These wellness shots are full of beneficial sirtuins and antioxidants, as well as a touch of olive oil which helps the body to absorb all the nutrients.

- Preparation Time: 0 minutes
- Cooking Time: 5 minutes
- Servings: 5

Ingredients:

- Turmeric root – 4 inches
- Ginger root – 4 inches
- Oranges, peeled – 2
- Lemons, peeled – 2
- Cayenne pepper - .125 teaspoon
- Black pepper, ground -.125 teaspoon
- Water - .75 cup
- Extra virgin olive oil - .5 teaspoon

Directions:

Pour the water into a boil. Once bubbling, add in the turmeric root and reduce the heat to a medium, allowing it to simmer for seven to eight minutes. Remove from the heat of the stove and take out the turmeric root, setting it aside. Pour the turmeric liquid into a container and let it chill in the fridge until cool.

While the turmeric liquid cools, run the ginger root, boiled turmeric root, oranges, and lemons, through your juicer.

Stir the turmeric liquid, seasonings, and oil into the prepared juice.

Enjoy a shot of this every morning. The leftover shots can keep in the fridge for two to three days.

Nutrition:

Kilocalories per Individual Serving 46

6. Iced Matcha Latte

You don't have to go to your local coffee shop or Starbucks to get a delicious iced matcha latte, you can make one at a fraction of the cost and without filler ingredients!

- Preparation Time: 0 minutes
- Cooking Time: 3 minutes
- Servings: 1

Ingredients:

- Matcha powder – 2 teaspoons
- Soy milk, unsweetened – 1 cup
- Hot water – 1.5 tablespoons
- Honey – 2 teaspoons

Directions:

Add the matcha and hot water to a bowl and whisk it until it is thoroughly combined without clumps. Ideally you want to use a bamboo matcha whisk in zigzag and circular formation.

In a glass over ice cubes add the soy milk and honey, stirring to combine. Slowly pour the matcha mixture over the top of the latte, lightly stirring it with a spoon. Serve immediately before the ice melts.

Nutrition:

Kilocalories per Individual Serving 123

7. Hot Matcha Latte

This matcha latte will warm you up in the winter and get your energy going all year long. While the ingredient is optional, adding in Maca root powder adds a wonderful flavor and health benefits to this beverage.

- Preparation Time: 0 minutes
- Cooking Time: 5 minutes
- Servings: 1

Ingredients:

- Matcha powder – 1.25 teaspoon
- Maca root powder - .25 teaspoon optional
- Hot water – 1 tablespoon
- Maple syrup – 1 tablespoon
- Soy milk, unsweetened – 1.5 cups

Directions:

Into a large mug add the matcha powder, Maca root, maple syrup, and hot water. Using a matcha bamboo whisk or standard kitchen whisk stir the ingredients together gently until the matcha and Maca have dissolved into the liquid. While I recommend using the matcha bamboo whisk, you can make do with whatever you have on hand.

Heat your soy milk, either in the microwave, on the stove, or with a steaming/frothing pitcher. While heating in the microwave is a quick option, I recommend using a steaming/frothing pitcher if you have one, or at the very least heating it on the stove. By heating on the stove you can use a whisk or a hand-held frothier to get the desired classic froth lattes usually have.

Pour the hot soy milk into the mug with the matcha, lightly stirring it to ensure the soy milk and matcha mixture have combined. Enjoy while hot.

Nutrition:

177 Kilocalories

8. Classic Latte with Cinnamon

This latte is a great way to increase your energy any time of the day! The flavors meld perfectly with a pinch of ground cinnamon, which is not only a great spice to add more flavor, but also an additional source of sirtuins.

- Preparation Time: 0 minutes
- Cooking Time: 5 minutes
- Servings: 1

Ingredients:

- Espresso – 2 ounces
- Soy milk, unsweetened – 10 ounces
- Date sugar – 1 teaspoon
- Cinnamon, ground - .25 teaspoon

Directions:

Heat your soy milk, either in the microwave, on the stove, or with a steaming/frothing pitcher. While heating in the microwave is a quick option, I recommend using a steaming/frothing pitcher if you have one, or at the very least heating it on the stove. By heating on the stove you can use a whisk or a handheld frothier to get the desired classic froth lattes usually have.

If your soy milk has developed a froth from whisking or using a frothier, then stir in the date sugar and cinnamon. However, if your soy milk hasn't developed a froth, then add the soy milk sugar, and cinnamon into a blender. Blend it for a minute, until it develops a dense froth.

Add your espresso to a mug and slowly pour the frothed milk over the top. Enjoy while warm.

Nutrition:

120 Kilocalories

9. Cold Brew Caramel Frappuccino

This Frappuccino takes preparation ahead of time to make the frozen soy milk cubes, cold brew coffee, and date caramel. But, it is worth it! You can easily keep these ingredients prepared ahead of time in your fridge or freezer so that you can make a delicious Frappuccino at a moment's notice.

- Preparation Time: 0 minutes
- Cooking Time: 10 minutes
- Servings: 2

Ingredients:

- Soy milk, unsweetened – 2 cups
- Coarsely ground dark coffee – 2 cups
- Filtered water – 4 cups
- Hot water – 3 tablespoons
- Pitted dates – 7
- Sea salt - .25 teaspoon

Directions:

Pour the unsweetened soy milk into an ice cube tray and freeze it overnight. Once frozen, use the cubes immediately or transfer them to a storage container so that they don't pick up flavors from the freezer.

Prepare the cold brew coffee overnight, as well. To do this, add the ground coffee and four cups of filtered water to a pitcher. Give the cold brew coffee a good stir, cover with a lid, and refrigerate overnight. The following day, strain the coffee through a fine mesh sieve or a coffee filter to remove the beans.

Pulse the pitted dates and sea salt with the hot water in a blender. You want to pulse until it forms a thick and smooth paste. Clean the sides of the blender with a spatula as needed. While this recipe calls for three tablespoons of hot water, you only want to use as much water as absolutely necessary. Therefore, slowly add the water, only adding as much as is needed to blend the dates into a smooth paste.

To prepare a single Frappuccino add half of the cold brew coffee, soy milk cubes, and date caramel until it forms a creamy drink. Serve!

Nutrition:

130 Kilocalories per Individual

Chapter 13 - Empowering Yourself with Sirt Foods

There are many uses and health benefits of Sirtfoods. Whether you are enjoying dark chocolate and wine or tofu and eggplant, you will find that you can enjoy these delicious ingredients in any meal or snack. We will be exploring the many health benefits these ingredients have to offer, along with some practical ways you can include them in your daily life. As you already know, Sirtfoods promote weight loss and weight management, so we will skip over these benefits and look toward other health benefits that they offer.

Buckwheat

Many people do not include buckwheat into their daily diets, but you should. Not only is it a great source of fiber, but it is also high in protein, and the carbohydrates will energize you when your calorie intake is limited. By adding in some buckwheat to your meals, you will help them stick with you longer, keeping you satisfied and energized longer than you otherwise would be. Another great bonus of buckwheat is that it is gluten-free, making it perfect for people with gluten intolerance or Celiac disease.

One cup U.S. system of measurement of cooked buckwheat contains more than 5.5 grams of protein, 4.5 grams of fiber, and 33.5 grams of carbohydrates. Along with these larger nutrients, they also contain important minerals such as potassium, magnesium, phosphorus, and calcium. Some vitamins found in buckwheat include vitamin K, B6, folate, niacin, thiamin, and riboflavin. As you already know, buckwheat is also high in antioxidant polyphenols sirtuins.

Buckwheat has been found to be a grain, or rather a pseudo cereal that is great for heart health. As we all should consider the health of our hearts while we age, we can all benefit from these benefits of buckwheat. Whole grains, such as buckwheat, are commonly recommended to be included in a person's daily diet to reduce heart disease. But, many people only eat refined grains, or if they are gluten-free may eat fewer grains altogether. Buckwheat is a great alternative to other grains, as it is typically eaten as a whole grain, it's rich in deep flavor, and studies have found it to stabilize blood pressure.

The high fiber content can also help in many ways. The fiber helps the gut to digest food more effectively, encouraging nutrient absorption, weight loss, and regularity. Fiber is also important in lowering cholesterol and therefore diseases associated with high cholesterol.

When using buckwheat, you can use either the grouts the hulled grain or flour. You can make pilaf, pancakes, soba noodles, crackers, porridge, fruit crumble, or even cookies

Dark Chocolate/Cocoa

A diet that allows chocolate? Yes! However, you can't mindlessly eat any variety or endless amounts of chocolate. While chocolate may be a great Sirtfood, its high in calories, meaning that excessive **Servings** can interfere with weight loss. Thankfully, since the Sirt diet manages calorie control, you shouldn't eat too much if you follow the guidelines. You should also stick with cocoa or dark chocolate 70% or higher. While milk and white chocolate may be delicious, they do not have the same health benefits.

One of the biggest benefits of dark chocolate is the role it plays in heart health. As many of the antioxidant sirtuins found within it are varieties especially helpful for heart health, you will find you can greatly reduce your risk of cardiovascular disease.

But, not only does the cocoa in dark chocolate reduce this harmful type of cholesterol, the cocoa butter in it has benefits, as well. Studies have shown that cocoa butter can increase HDL good cholesterol. This is great news, as HDL cholesterol is helpful for heart health, as it removes bad cholesterol from the bloodstream.

While it may sound contradictory to say eating sweets can help prevent diabetes, and while that may be contradictory if you were to make such claims about milk or white chocolate, chocolate does have this anti-diabetic effect. This is because the chocolate actually changes the way your body metabolizes glucose. When both of these effects are combined, it greatly reduces your risk of developing diabetes or can even manage your condition in conjunction with your doctor's treatment.

Do you ever feel happier after eating chocolate? It's not just from enjoying a sweet treat, as studies have proven dark chocolate to have a beneficial effect on mental health! The reason for this is because chocolate activates the neurons in your brain associated with reward and pleasure while decreasing the stress response. Along with boosting your moods, these studies have also found that chocolate can improve cognition and memory.

Of course, you can eat dark chocolate plain or make healthy versions of popular sweets with it, but you can also use it in savory food! Try adding some cocoa to a pot of chili to increase flavor depth, to meat marinades and rubs, into mole that can be used to complement a number of Latino dishes, or even to a sweet-savory salad.

Coffee

You may only think of coffee as a necessity to stay awake, or worse; you might even consider it an unhealthy addiction. However, just like tea has health benefits, so too does coffee. In a single cup of coffee, you can get plenty of vitamins B2, B3, B5, potassium, and manganese.

Not only does coffee cause the breakdown of fat to being a Sirt food, but it can also increase your physical performance allowing your workouts to be more effective. Studies have found that the consumption of coffee leads to a performance increase of twelve percent, so try to drink a strong cup half an hour prior to your workout.

People who drink coffee experience a significantly reduced risk of developing diabetes. Studies have found that depending on a person's coffee consumption; they can reduce their likelihood of developing the disease by twenty-three to sixty-seven percent. With each cup, you drink your risk drops by seven percent. However, you should keep in mind that it's important to stay within recommended daily **Servings**, which is three to five cups. Of course, your doctor will know if you have to alter this daily intake depending on your individual health, so ask them for their input.

Depression is a severe mental illness, which is one of the most common causes of disability in the United States. While it's hard to understand how severe the condition is if you haven't suffered from it yourself, those who have to know just how debilitating it is, Depression makes it hard just to get out of bed each day, just to stay alive. Yet, many people are quietly suffering without ever seeking help. Thankfully, coffee can help. Many people use coffee and chocolate to reduce symptoms, which, in conjunction with prescribed medication, can increase the quality of life. A study by Harvard found that when people drink four or more cups a day, they experienced a twenty percent reduced risk of being depressed. In another study, it was found when people drink four or more cups a day; they are fifty-three percent less likely to commit suicide.

Coffee can be added to sweet or savory dishes, such as meat rubs and marinades, chili, mole and barbecue sauces, roasted root vegetables, red-eye gravy, or even salad vinaigrette.

Medjool Dates

Grown in the tropics, most of the dates you find in Western countries are the dried variety. They are highly sweet and chewy and are sometimes even sold in the form of date sugar to be used in baked goods, coffee, or anything else you might want to sweeten. This is beneficial, as coconut palm sugar has more health benefits than cane sugar.

A standard three and a half ounce serving of dates contains plenty of fiber, magnesium, potassium, iron, copper, manganese, and vitamin B6.

A large amount of fiber in the fruit is great for your digestive health. It can help to slow down digestion so that you better absorb nutrients from your food while also making you more regular. Another reason fiber is important is because it reduces the likelihood of blood sugar spikes and manages blood glucose levels.

Preliminary studies have found dates to lower inflammation in the brain, which can reduce the risk of Alzheimer's and Parkinson's disease, along with other neurodegenerative disorders. It can also reduce Alzheimer's by reducing plaque that forms in the brain.

Sugar can be added to a number of savory dishes to balance out flavors, and you can add date sugar in these dishes instead. Try adding some date sugar to a bowl of buckwheat porridge, to teriyaki sauce, or even to salads.

Kale

Kale is categorized as a calciferous vegetable, is a member of the cabbage family, and is considered one of the most nutritionally-dense foods on earth. A single cup serving of ale contains large numbers of vitamins K, A, C, and B6, along with the minerals manganese, copper, calcium, magnesium, and potassium. All of this nutrition is packed in only thirty-three calories, making it a great choice to add to your daily diet.

The vitamin C in kale is widely known to strengthen the immune system and ward off illness, but that is not all. For instance, vitamin C is a vital component necessary for the synthesis of collagen in the body. Collagen is an essential aspect of whole-body health, as it makes up our organs, skin, and bones. Kale is one of the best vegetables for vitamin C consumption, and it has even more than an orange. But, know that when heat is applied to vitamin C it is destroyed, so if you want to reap the benefits of this vitamin, enjoy your kale raw.

Vitamin K, while being an important nutrient, is often under-consumed. Thankfully, you can consume all of your needed daily vitamin K, and then some, in a single serving of kale. By doing this, you can ensure your blood clots perfectly and that it is able to utilize the calcium you consume.

Kale is able to reduce cholesterol by containing a substance known as bile acid sequestrates. Naturally, this lowered cholesterol reduces a person's risk of heart attack and cardiovascular diseases.

Along with salads and green juice, you can also try making crispy kale chips, savory kale sautés, or add it into pasta, grain dishes, soups, and casseroles.

Conclusion

Sirtfoods are practically all sound decisions and may even bring about some medical advantages because of their cancer prevention agent or calming properties.

However eating only a bunch of especially solid nourishments can't meet the entirety of your body's wholesome needs.

The Sirtfood Diet is superfluously prohibitive and offers no unmistakable, special medical advantages over some other sort of diet.

Moreover, eating just 1,000 calories is normally not suggested without the supervision of a doctor. In any event, eating 1,500 calories for each day is unreasonably prohibitive for some individuals.

The diet likewise requires drinking up to three green juices for each day. Despite the fact that juices can be a decent wellspring of nutrients and minerals, they are additionally a wellspring of sugar and contain practically none of the solid fiber that entire foods grown from the ground do.

Likewise, tasting on juice all through the entire day is a poorly conceived notion for both your glucose and your teeth.

Also, in light of the fact that the diet is so restricted in calories and nourishment decision, it is more than likely insufficient in protein, nutrients and minerals, particularly during the main stage.

Because of the low calorie levels and prohibitive nourishment decisions, this diet might be difficult to adhere to for the whole three weeks.

Add that to the high starting expenses of buying a juicer, the guide and certain uncommon and costly fixings, just as the time expenses of getting ready specific suppers and juices, and this diet gets unfeasible and impractical for some individuals.

The Sirtfood Diet advances solid nourishments however is prohibitive in calories and nourishment decisions. It additionally includes drinking bunches of juice, which is anything but a sound suggestion.

Despite the fact that the main period of the Sirtfood Diet is exceptionally low in calories and healthfully inadequate, there are no genuine wellbeing worries for the normal, sound grown-up thinking about the diet's brief term.

However for somebody with diabetes, calorie limitation and drinking generally squeeze for the initial scarcely any days of the diet may cause risky changes in glucose levels.

In any case, even a sound individual may encounter some reactions — principally hunger.

Eating just 1,000–1,500 calories for each day will leave pretty much anybody feeling hungry, particularly if quite a bit of what you're expending is juice, which is low in fiber, a supplement that helps keep you feeling full.

During stage one, you may encounter opposite reactions, for example, weakness, discombobulating and fractiousness because of the calorie limitation.

For the generally sound grown-up, genuine wellbeing results are far-fetched if the diet is followed for just three weeks.

It might leave you hungry, yet it's not perilous for the normal sound grown-up.

The Bottom Line

The Sirtfood Diet is loaded with sound nourishments, however not smart dieting designs.

Also, its hypothesis and wellbeing claims depend on terrific extrapolations from starter scientific proof.

Adding sirtfoods to your diet is certifiably not a poorly conceived notion and may significantly offer some medical advantages, the diet itself looks like simply one more prevailing fashion.

Set aside yourself the cash and jump to making energizing, long haul dietary changes.

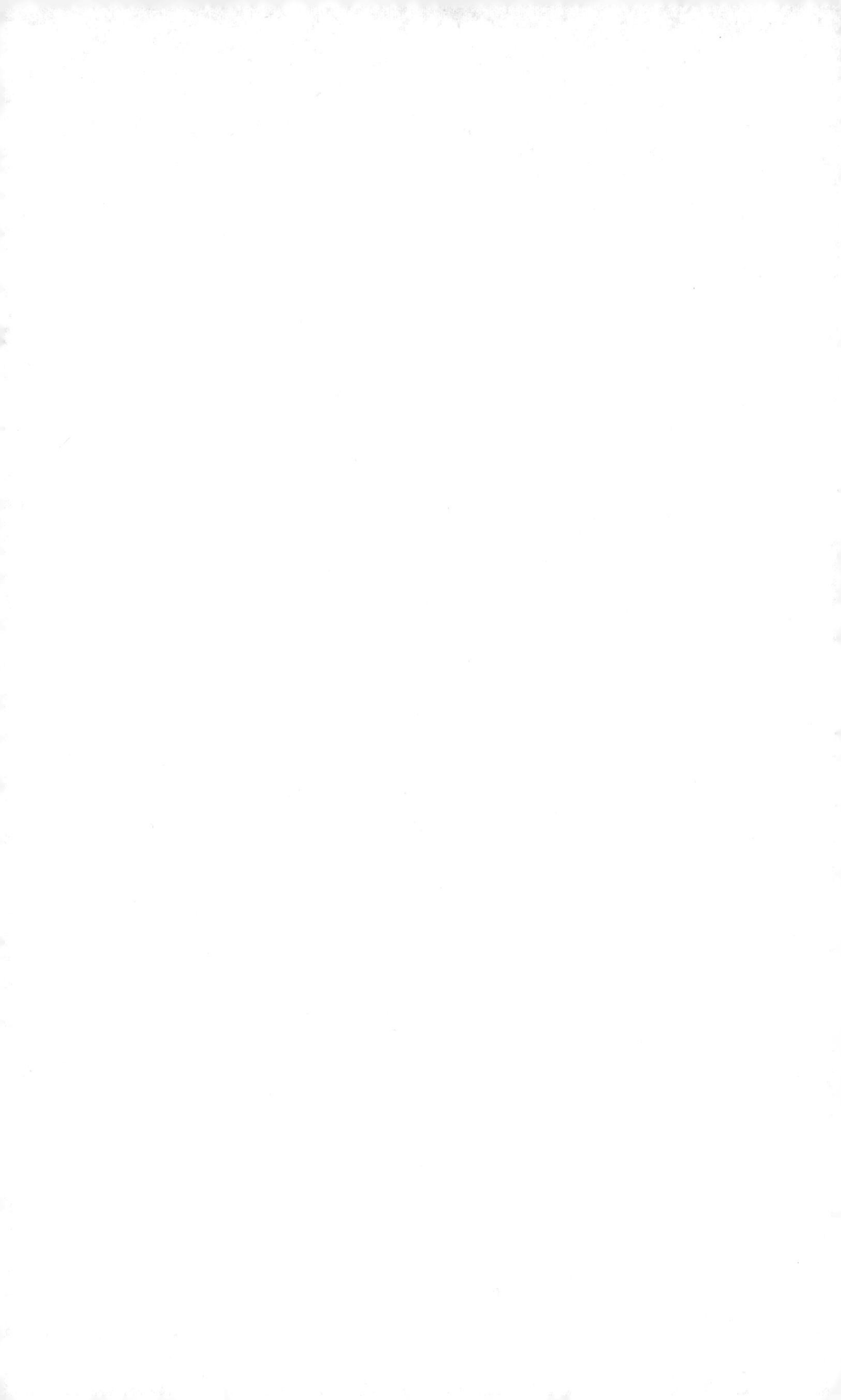